THE SECRET OF VITAMIN D:

How to Detect a Vitamin D Deficiency and Easily Reverse It.

Don C. Allen

Table of contents

Introduction

Unfortunately, according to scientists, almost a billion individuals worldwide lack enough vitamin D. You probably aren't aware of the fact that vitamin D isn't a vitamin. It is a prohormone.

A substance known as a prohormone is one that your body will convert into a hormone. In contrast to other vitamins, this prohormone has receptors on every cell in your body. We shall refer to this prohormone by its most popular name, vitamin D, for convenience.

A prohormone must be converted into a form that your body can utilize. When this occurs, vitamin D circulates throughout your body and serves several purposes. It is essential for strong bones and supports bone growth as well as the well-being of your muscles.

In this special report, we'll cover why vitamin D is so crucial for your health, what causes vitamin D insufficiency and its warning signs, as well as what you can do to maintain healthy levels of vitamin D in your body.

The benefits of vitamin D on your body

Vitamin D is crucial for strong bones, as we discussed in the opening. Strong bones are developed as a result, which is crucial as you become older. Additionally, calcium from your blood will be taken up by vitamin D, which will then be used to build and repair bone and muscle tissue. For the parathyroid gland to effectively control the levels of calcium in your blood, you also need vitamin D.

Deficiencies in vitamin D

The most prevalent kind of vitamin D deficiency is known as "rickets," which you may have heard of previously. Children that don't properly mineralize their bone tissue may have rickets. Their bones typically become excessively soft as a result, becoming malformed.

But rickets is not the only condition caused by a lack of vitamin D. Numerous other health issues might arise from a vitamin D shortage, according to numerous research. These topics will be covered later in this special report.

Additionally essential to your immune system is vitamin D. Each of your immune cells has a receptor for vitamin D, and they can produce the active hormone or metabolite of vitamin D. This proves that there is unquestionably a link between them.

Additionally, autoimmune diseases including multiple sclerosis and rheumatoid arthritis are linked to vitamin D deficiency. Your immune system will work properly and guard you against autoimmune diseases and other infections when the appropriate level of vitamin D is present in your blood.

For your body to communicate, you need vitamin D.

Your body needs to have the right amount of calcium, and vitamin D will work with your skeleton, kidneys, and intestines to make sure this is the case. Your body needs the right amounts of calcium for healthy and strong bones.

Your parathyroid gland will take calcium from your skeleton if there is not enough calcium for your bones or if your vitamin D levels are inadequate, which weakens your bones overall.

We shall talk about the root reasons for vitamin D insufficiency in the section after this.

Why Is Vitamin D Deficiency Occurring?

There are several reasons why people lack vitamin D. The fundamental issue is that it's not always simple to identify a vitamin D deficiency. To identify it, you must be aware of the symptoms. This likely explains why researchers estimate that more than a billion people worldwide have vitamin D deficiencies.

In further detail, we'll go over vitamin D deficiency symptoms in the following section. We will examine some of the most typical reasons for vitamin D insufficiency in this article.

Your diet may contribute to a vitamin D deficiency.

You may become vitamin D deficient if you don't consume the foods that promote the production of vitamin D. Animal-based foods that support vitamin D development include:

- Fish Beef liver
- Egg yolk
- Fish oil
- Enhanced milk products

Since vegans do not eat any of these items, they are more likely to get vitamin D deficiencies. Vegans who want to make up for the vitamin D they are missing out on can take supplements.

Your skin is dark.

If you have dark skin, the pigment, or melanin, may stop vitamin D from forming when you are exposed to sunlight. This is true whether you are naturally dark-skinned or have a tan.

The simple line is that the less likely it is for your skin to produce vitamin D when exposed to direct sunshine, the darker you are. This can be a problem even if you spend a lot of time in the sun.

Your Digestive Tract is Giving You Trouble

Some patients have digestive system issues, which prevent them from absorbing dietary fat or vitamin D. An illness like cystic fibrosis, celiac disease, or Crohn's disease may make it more difficult for your intestines to absorb the vitamin D you eat.

Because vitamin D is fat-soluble, these medical problems can also limit the absorption of dietary fats, which can lead to the same issue.

You do not receive sufficient sunlight.

Only when you are exposed to direct sunshine does your skin begin to produce vitamin D. You are far more likely to be vitamin D deficient if you don't spend a lot of time outside.

You can be confined to your home or have a profession that keeps you from obtaining much sunlight. Living in a northern latitude country can make it difficult to get adequate sunshine. For religious reasons, wearing robes and head coverings might reduce exposure to the sun.

Living somewhere with a lot of pollution or smog might also limit your exposure to sunshine. The place you reside, the time of year, and the day of the week that you spend outside in the sun can all have a significant impact. Due to the sun's position and the ozone layer, some regions of the US, including Cleveland, Ohio, will experience no UV-B light for six months out of the year. Please be advised that the sun is at its peak strength from 10 am to 3 pm.

You are obese or overweight.

Having excess body fat or being obese can lead to vitamin D deficiency. Your fat cells might not be effective enough to draw the necessary amount of vitamin D from your blood and distribute it throughout your body if you have a body mass index of 30 or higher.

Vitamin D cannot be effectively processed by your kidneys.

Your kidneys are crucial in transforming vitamin D into its active form. Your kidneys may be unable to carry out the conversion process adequately, leading to a vitamin D deficiency, if they are damaged, sick, or have slowed down with age.

You're Getting Older

As we age, it becomes more challenging for our skin to produce vitamin D from sunlight. There may be enough vitamin D in your blood, but your kidneys are unable to convert it as effectively as they once could because as you age, your kidneys also tend to slow down.

You use Particular Drugs

Unfortunately, several drugs have the potential to cause vitamin D insufficiency. If you use laxatives, there's a chance that the vitamin D and other nutrients will be washed out of your system before you can absorb them. Steroid use can also be problematic since it tends to limit calcium absorption, which interferes with vitamin D metabolism.

Since cholesterol is a source of vitamin D, using drugs to lower cholesterol, like colestipol or satins, can cause your body to produce less vitamin D.

The levels of vitamin D absorption in your body might be decreased by some weight reduction medications like orlistat. Taking seizure medicine like phenobarbital and phenytoin might also have an impact on your body's levels of vitamin D. Furthermore, thiazide diuretics like indapamide and HCTZ (hydrochlorothiazide) will often reduce urinary calcium excretion. Hypercalcemia may occur if you use vitamin D supplements along with certain thiazide drugs.

We'll talk about the signs of vitamin D deficiency in the following part.

Symptoms of Vitamin D Deficiency

There are not many trustworthy vitamin D deficiency symptoms, so we advise that you visit your doctor and get a blood test done. However, there are a few signs of vitamin D inadequacy that you should be aware of.

Having cramps, feeling weak, or having achy muscles

A study was conducted with volunteers who had experienced chronic pain. According to the study, more than 70% of the subjects had a vitamin D deficiency. Your body contains some vitamin D receptors on nociceptors that detect pain. Vitamin D deficiency has been linked to sensitivity and pain in another mouse study.

Taking vitamin D supplements has aided people with chronic pain, according to other human studies. Always remember that aches and pains are your body's way of telling you that something is amiss.

You Experience Constant Fatigue

Chronic fatigue syndrome may indicate a vitamin D insufficiency. Visit your doctor and request a blood test if you constantly feel exhausted. Please keep in mind that other issues might lead to chronic tiredness besides vitamin D deficiency.

Frequently Contracting Infections

Your body's immune system cells that assist in warding off infections require direct interaction with vitamin D. According to numerous studies, there is a connection between a vitamin D deficiency and respiratory tract illnesses such as pneumonia, influenza, bronchitis, and the common cold.

Again, if you think you have too many illnesses, visit your doctor and request a blood test to determine whether you are vitamin D deficient.

Bone and lower back pain

You may be significantly vitamin D deficient if you experience lower back discomfort or pain in your bones. It can also indicate that you've had a long-term vitamin D deficiency.

A large loss of calcium from bone tissue causes lower back or bone discomfort. It takes time for this calcium to form. Visit your physician for a blood test if you are feeling these pains.

The Healing Process for Wounds Is Protracted

According to studies done in test tubes, vitamin D increases your body's levels of the chemicals that help heal wounds by forming new skin.

In other investigations, it was discovered that subjects with lower vitamin D levels are more likely to have higher levels of inflammatory markers. These are known to impede the correct functioning of the healing process and slow it down. If your wounds take a while to heal, ask your doctor about a blood test.

You've Got Hair Loss

More often in women than in males, this is an indication of vitamin D deficiency. You should be aware that there is now little solid scientific evidence to substantiate the association between vitamin D insufficiency and female hair loss.

An autoimmune condition called alopecia areata causes severe hair loss on the head and other parts of the body. There is a connection to rickets, which is known to be caused by a lack of vitamin D in children. Visit your doctor for a blood test to assess your vitamin D levels if you are balding.

You Observe Mood Shifts

This is a fascinating symptom because tests on some depressed people revealed low levels of vitamin D, which raises the intriguing question of why depression is associated with vitamin D deficiency. The good news is that the depression slightly lessened when these patients treated their vitamin D deficiency.

We will talk about the potential effects of vitamin D deficiency in the next section.

Possible Consequences of Vitamin D Deficiency

You may have a wide range of issues if your vitamin D levels are low. The most typical issues that people with low vitamin D levels may have are covered in this section.

Heart disease with elevated blood pressure

A lack of vitamin D has been linked to high blood pressure, strokes, peripheral artery disease (PAD), congestive heart failure, and heart disease, according to numerous studies.

According to studies, having the proper quantities of vitamin D in your body also helps to control renal blood pressure.

Bone disorders and Osteoporosis

Your body's bones are constantly being reshaped. Your bones will break down more quickly as you age than they will build up. For women who are going through menopause, this is especially true. As you become older, your bone density decreases.

Osteoporosis can be brought on by chronic calcium or vitamin D insufficiency. Your muscles need vitamin D for proper growth and development, and your bones depend on those muscles for support.

Autoimmune Conditions

Numerous autoimmune diseases, including systemic lupus erythematosus, inflammatory bowel disease, rheumatoid arthritis, and multiple sclerosis, are linked to vitamin D insufficiency, according to mounting research.

Vitamin D levels are typically lower in patients with certain autoimmune illnesses than in healthy individuals.

Problems during Pregnancy

A 2019 study found a connection between vitamin deficiencies and pregnant women who were at risk for preeclampsia, which can lead to premature delivery. A possible connection between a vitamin D deficiency and gestational diabetes was also raised by the study.

Vitamin D deficiency during pregnancy increases the risk of developing bacterial vaginosis. You should be aware that getting too much vitamin D during pregnancy may increase the risk of a kid having food allergies in the first two years of life.

Higher Infection Risk

Before the development of antibiotics, the treatment for some infections, such as tuberculosis, included taking cod liver oil every day and exposing the patient to a lot of sunlight. Numerous studies have suggested a connection between a lack of vitamin D and an increase in infections.

The Diabetes Risk

The pancreas' ability to control blood sugar levels is one of vitamin D's most crucial roles. Additionally, vitamin D tends to increase your body's sensitivity to insulin. Your body produces this hormone to control your blood sugar levels. Diabetes may develop as a result of insulin resistance brought on by a vitamin D deficiency.

The Cancer Types' Risk

The proper amounts of vitamin D in your body will aid in preventing the growth of any abnormal cells in breast or colon tissues. This may also aid in the treatment of disorders like breast or colon cancer. Prostate cancer may potentially be prevented with vitamin D.

We will talk about foods that contain vitamin D in the next section.

Food sources of vitamin D

Minerals and vitamins are frequently added to processed foods these days. The bulk of dairy products and some cereals are frequently fortified with vitamin D.

The animal items with the highest vitamin D content include fatty fish and cow liver (e.g.

mackerel, salmon, and tuna). International units are used to measure the amount of vitamin D in meals (IU).

Vitamin D Content of Particular Foods

From lowest to highest, the following foods are listed according to their vitamin D content:

Veggies and fruits - Grains and Cereals with No IU Portabella mushrooms have no IU; half a cup has 4 IU Swiss cheese; one ounce has 6 IU Cheddar cheese; one ounce has 12 IU fortified cereal; one cup has 40 IU egg yolk; one large yolk has 41 IU cooked beef liver; three ounces has 42 IU for scrambled eggs; one large egg has 44 IU for sardines (in a can with oil drained); two sardines have 46 IU for

This list demonstrates that some animal products contain higher levels of vitamin D than other diets. When you go grocery shopping, look at the nutrition labels to determine how much of the desired products contain vitamin D. Be cautious as foods that have been fortified may not always have the same levels of vitamin D.

You require how much vitamin D

Your age will determine how much vitamin D you need daily if you are in excellent health. You will need to ingest more vitamin D as you age since your body won't be able to produce and use as much vitamin D as it does when you're younger.

We will give you the recommended daily allowances (RDA) for vitamin D for each age group in this section. You should be aware that if you currently have a deficit or are at risk of developing bone problems like osteoporosis, your doctor may advise you to eat higher quantities of vitamin D. Make an appointment to talk about your needs with your doctor.

Recommended Daily Amounts (RDA) of Vitamin D by Age Group

Please pay close attention to the list's upper bounds. Being a fat-soluble vitamin, vitamin D overdose can result in hazardous accumulation in the body.

- Avoid exceeding the daily recommendations for vitamin D without your doctor's approval as doing so can have dangerous negative effects.

- infants under six months old need 400 IU per day (do not exceed 1,000 IU per day)
- infants aged 6 to 12 months need 400 IU each day (do not exceed 1,500 IU per day)
- Children aged 1-3 years old need 600 IU each day (do not exceed 2,500 IU per day)
- Children aged 4 to 8 need 600 IU each day (do not exceed 3,000 IU per day)
- Adults and children over the age of nine need 600 IU each day (do not exceed 4,000 IU per day)
- Adults above the age of 70 need 800 IU each day (do not exceed 4,000 IU per day)
- Women between the ages of 14 and 50 who are pregnant or nursing need 600 IU each day (do not exceed 4,000 IU per day)

We'll talk about diagnosing and treating a vitamin D shortage in the following section.

Treatment and Diagnosis of Vitamin D Deficiency

To determine whether you are vitamin D deficient, you should first speak with your doctor. You won't need to fast before the test or prepare in any other way; your doctor will simply draw some blood. A 25-hydroxyvitamin D test is typically used by doctors to check for vitamin D insufficiency.

You should be aware that this blood test is distinct from the one you could have at a routine physical. Make sure to tell your doctor that you are worried you might not be getting enough vitamin D.

Most healthy people consider the test results good if they reveal that your blood has between 20 and 50 nanograms of vitamin D per milliliter (ng/ml).

The doctor will tell you that you are vitamin D deficient if the result is less than 12 to 20 ng/ml. Your doctor will advise you to take a supplement or eat foods high in vitamin D each day.

Your physician might recommend varying amounts of vitamin D

To raise your vitamin D levels to the suggested range we previously described, your doctor may prescribe vitamin D levels that are greater than those levels.

Instead of advising you to eat foods like fortified milk products, beef liver, or fish, which have a higher vitamin D concentration, your doctor is likely to recommend a supplement.

Different Vitamin D Types

You should be aware that there are two varieties of vitamin D: D2 and D3. Cholecalciferol, or D2, is a substance that is present in animal products. Ergocalciferol, generally known as vitamin D3, is a substance that some plants contain.

Most pharmacies sell D3 over the counter. A prescription is necessary for D2 if your doctor recommends it. D2 is often sold in doses of 50,000 IU, which you will take once or twice per week. Your body can absorb D3 more quickly.

Limit your intake of vitamin D.

You can never get too much vitamin D from exposure to sunlight. However, taking supplements makes it simple to overdose on vitamin D, which can have unpleasant side effects like hypercalcemia (excess calcium in the blood), poor appetite, constipation, increased thirst, and urination, or nausea.

Extreme vitamin D overdoses can result in ataxia, weakness, and confusion (this is a neurological issue that can make you slur your words and act clumsily).

You should be on the lookout for these symptoms if your doctor prescribes a higher dosage of vitamin D, and you should let your doctor know right away if you do.

Avoid taking too much vitamin A

Keep an eye on your vitamin A intake in addition to your vitamin D intake. Similar to vitamin D, excess vitamin A in the body can build up and have harmful negative effects.

Conclusion

In the US, many people do not consume the required daily allowance of vitamin D. Approximately 92% of males and over 97% of girls (an average of 94% of all persons) over a year old received less than the recommended daily quantity of 400 IU from the food they consumed, according to a three-year study from 2013 to 2016 by the National Health and Nutrition Examination Survey.

The average daily intake of vitamin D through food and drink was found to be roughly 204 IU in men and just 168 IU in women, according to further study of this data. Only 196 IU was given to kids between the ages of 2 and 19 daily.

Approximately 28% of individuals over the age of two, 26% of people between the ages of 2 and 5, and 14% of participants between the ages of 6 and 11 all reported supplement use, according to the data.

With age, more people began using supplements. 10% of individuals between the ages of 12 and 19 took supplements, and 49% of men and 59% of women over 60 also did so.

It should come as no surprise that the study also found that eating a healthy diet significantly raised participants' levels of vitamin D. Consuming a variety of fruits, vegetables, whole grains, low-fat or fat-free milk products, and healthy oils constitutes a healthy diet in the United States.

drinking milk, eating cereals, yogurt, margarine, and vitamin D-fortified orange juice. Cheese contains trace quantities of vitamin D.

Protein-rich foods to eat include soy products, seeds, nuts, legumes, eggs, poultry, lean meat, and seafood.

Consume fatty fish like tuna, salmon, and mackerel, since they are all excellent sources of vitamin D. Vitamin D levels are lower in beef liver and egg yolks.

Reduce your consumption of saturated and trans fats.

Limit your intake of added sweets and sodium.

The point being made is obvious. To prevent a vitamin D deficiency, eat foods high in vitamin

D and spend time outside in the sun. Check with your doctor if you believe you may be vitamin D deficient.

www.ingramcontent.com/pod-product-compliance
Lightning Source LLC
Chambersburg PA
CBHW061646130726
47996CB00003B/1483

Everything You Need to Know About Social Anxiety Disorder

Causes ◆ Symptoms ◆ Treatment

Watch a video version:
https://www.youtube.com/watch?v=tdPaDcFSn_Q

This book is based on information and recommendations by the Department of Health, United States government.

Created By The Bizmove Health Team

Disclaimer

All the content found in this book was created for informational purposes only. The Content is not intended to be a substitute for professional medical advice, diagnosis, or treatment. Always seek the advice of your physician or other qualified health provider with any questions you may have regarding a medical condition. Never disregard professional medical advice or delay in seeking it because of something you have read in this book.